SHIELA DUGGAN

4 Habits To Lose Weight

Follow the Steps for a New Healthy Lifestyle

First edition

This book was professionally typeset on Reedsy.
Find out more at reedsy.com

Contents

1

Introduction

Welcome to 4 Habits To Lose Weight guide. My name is Shiela Duggan. I would like to take you to my journey that got me the result at age 45 and have kept the weight off.

If you are like me, after college, life got busy. I got a job, got married, had a family, was busy with my social life and my "ME" time was not a priority. Before you know it, my clothes stopped fitting. Then I started exploring different types of diet, from protein shakes or meal replacements, to buying meal plans, signing up for classes at the gym and then quitting midway. Yes, it would work at first, then as soon as I stopped, I would gain the weight back plus more. It was like that for me for 15 years. I was on a Yo-yo diet. I get so motivated at the beginning of the year then I get bored and would just go back to my lifestyle because I could not give up on my social life or would refuse to sacrifice sweets, snacks, alcohol, and carbs.

I thought I could motivate myself and say I can do it, and every year when New Year's comes along, I would sign up for a different program because in my mind, this year is going to be different. I can do it. Then midway, I would stop again because for whatever it is, life gets hectic.

I would compare myself to everyone else. The questions that come to mind: How do they do it all? How do they have time for themselves? What are they doing to look that good? I would then answer myself and make the excuse why it does not work for me i.e. They do not have any kids, no job, they do not have a busy schedule like I do. The list would go on and on. I was validating to myself that it is okay to fall off because they do not have my hectic schedule.

Every year, my New Year's resolution will include "lose weight." So, for 15 years, I kept doing the same thing over and over. The worst part for me, after I hit forty, my metabolism slowed down more. All the weight was shifting from different areas of my body. I would also have mood swings and night sweats. Then speaking with my Dr. I am going through perimenopause. My body was going through a lot of hormonal changes. So, it is getting worse as I age.

One day, I was looking at myself in the mirror and saw my belly fat! I was mortified. My thoughts: I destroyed my body by having two kids. It is time to accept that this is how my body will be. I am a mommy now. Come to terms with my new "ME" and adjust accordingly. I started wearing those long sweaters on top of my shirt just to minimize the "I'm getting fat look." I started layering or whatever I can do just to hide the fact that I have gained weight. Then when I am taking photos, I would make sure I am behind someone else. I started asking myself questions. How much more can I hide? How did I get here? How can I turn this around? If they can do it, I can do it too. These were the same questions that I would ask myself over and over.

Last year, almost 45 years old, my Dr. told me that my cholesterol keeps going up and if I cannot control it, she would need me to start taking medication. This is when reality hits me. My family has a history of heart disease, and I do not want anything to happen to me at an early age, especially with 2 kids. I want to live a long life. I want to see them get married and see my grandchildren someday. This is when I found a new purpose in life. I was determined to make a change and do whatever it takes to get to my goal. It is time for "ME" time.

So, where do I begin? This is when I realized, I must be in the right mindset to make this happen. I want to be healthy again before I hit 50. I want to feel good, look good and show my kids that their mom will be there for them for a long haul but to do that, I must carve out time for myself. This New Year's resolution does not say "lose weight," instead I wrote down "self-care." I am determined to make this work for my family.

So, I started my journey of getting my body back and starting the road to being healthy! My 4 habits that I incorporated made an enormous difference for me and I can finally say, I found something that has kept my weight off for a year and counting. I am much happier, more energetic and the best part, my kids have been watching me for a year and they also try to be a part of my daily routine. I hope this book will also give you confidence that you CAN do it too. I cannot wait to share it with you. I know if you follow my daily regimen, you too will get GREAT RESULTS.

DOUBT

2

First Habit: Intermittent Fasting

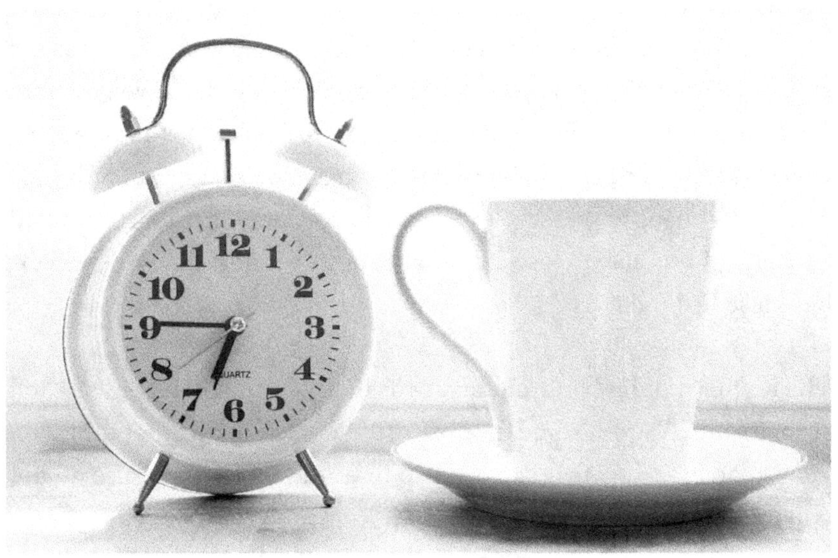

What is intermittent fasting you ask? I did not know anything about it either until a friend told me it works. Intermittent fasting is when you choose to go without food for a set period of time. For me, I use the 16-

8 method: Fast for 16 hours and you select your 8 hours eating window. My schedule is 12PM - 8PM daily. I am not much of a breakfast person, so these times work for me. You can choose your time that works for you. There are of course several types of methods (12- 12, 5 - 12, the alternate days method and 24 hours method), but 16 - 8 is the most common use.

Before you start freaking out that you cannot do it, there are benefits of intermittent fasting. It helps with hormonal dis balance and helps maintain proper hormone levels. Additionally, it can help burn fat.

As I got older, I started noticing that my metabolism is slowing down, it is harder for me to lose body fat and as I go through perimenopause. My body is going through a lot of hormonal changes. Since I started the intermittent fasting, I saw changes right away. I do not have the night sweats as much and I am sleeping better, and my body fat is disappearing slowly. Yes, it was hard at first but to form a habit you must do this for 21 days. So, hang in there, you will be glad you did. Once I incorporated this habit, I was able to lose 8lbs in a month. Not only did I lose weight, but I also lost inches.

The best part of intermittent fasting is that you cook fewer meals and clean up less. You get some time back for yourself to do other things on your to do list. Now that I am used to intermittent fasting, I also do not crave all the food that I used to eat.

I also try to be busy so that I am not thinking about food. I find that the busier I am, the less I crave the things I used to eat.

Please check with your healthcare provider if intermittent fasting is right for you. Discuss the pros and cons. It is of course not recommended for women that are pregnant or breastfeeding, underweight, take medicine for diabetes or low blood sugar.

3

Second Habit: Drink Plenty of Fluids

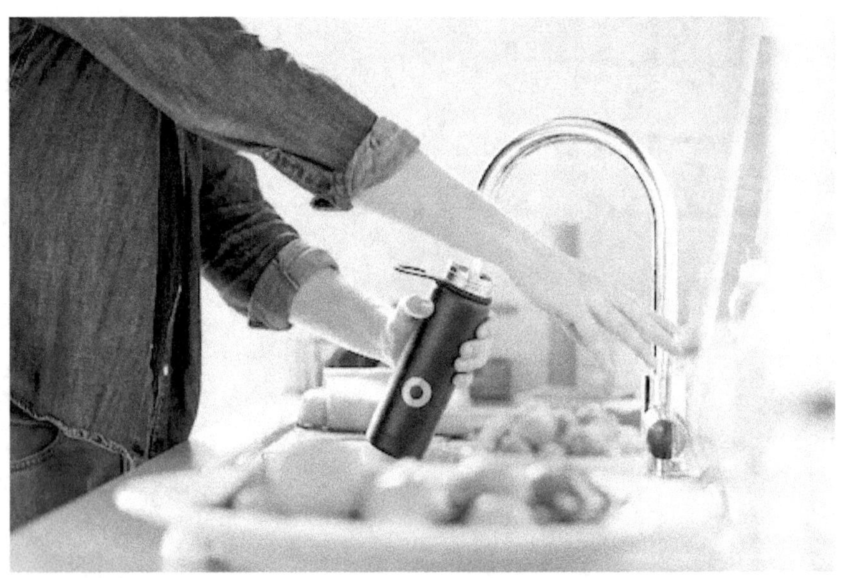

I drink about a gallon of fluids a day. Before I did anything, I made a habit that I would drink a cup of water first thing in the morning. I would use a splash of Mio and 1 tablespoon of Apple Cider Vinegar (ACV Brand: Bragg) and mix it with a cup of hot water. I like mine warm, so it feels like I am drinking tea. It is not for everyone, but I do not mind the taste. Note: Do not take ACV by itself. It is hard on your teeth, it can weaken your tooth enamel. I recommend mixing it with water or sparkling water and a splash of Mio. Throughout the day I drink water. I have a jug that measures my water intake so I can make sure I am on track. Continuous water intake also helps me curve my appetite, so I am not as hungry. Occasionally, I would drink black coffee or tea or flavored sparkling water. If you are drinking coffee or tea, do not add any dairy, cream, or sugar.

Now, why do I add Apple Cider Vinegar to my drinks? It is because of the benefits that it offers. Due to my cholesterol concern, I know it regulates bad cholesterol and high blood pressure. It breaks down fat and helps you accelerate your weight loss. It heals your skin and reverses the sign of aging that is caused by overexposure to the sun. These are some of the benefits, but I know there are so much more benefits to incorporating ACV to your daily routine. I drink my ACV first thing in the morning and before I go to bed.

I know a lot of people cannot drink only plain water or plain coffee without adding dairy or sugar or other supplements. If you cut sugar and dairy from your diet, you will see a significant difference at the end of 8 weeks. You can add lemon or mint or cucumber in your water for added flavor or try La Croix sparkling water, especially the Limoncello flavor. Try other flavors too. Get something that would satisfy your palette. So go ahead and experiment with assorted flavors but no sugar added or dairy and your goal is a gallon of water a day.

There are benefits of drinking water. It helps us hydrate. Helps with weight loss. Great for your skin. It also helps you build your muscles and is good for your joints.

Drinking a gallon of water will help flush out your system. If you are not used to drinking water, keep trying and push yourself to consume the gallon goal a day, your body will thank you later. I know it may not happen overnight but if you incorporate it daily it will soon stick, and you will not even think twice later.

Third Habit: Exercise

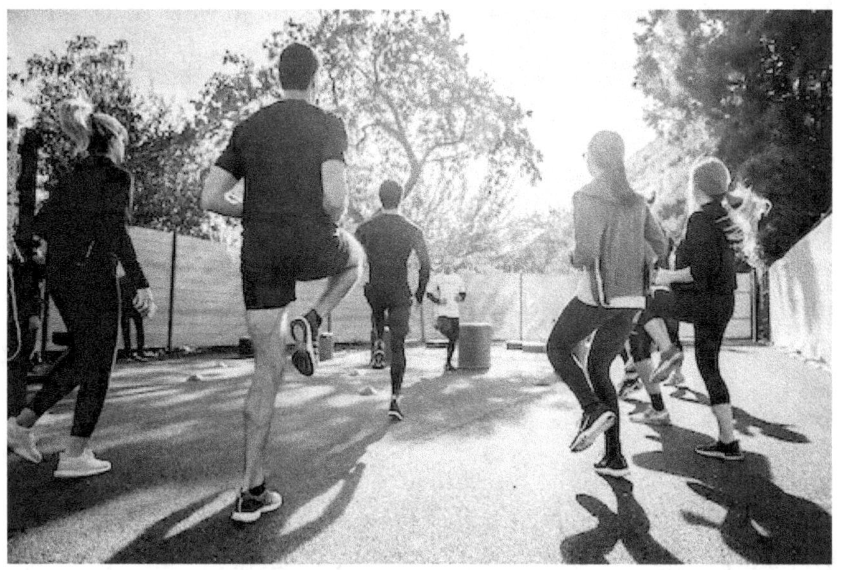

Exercise is the hardest thing for me to incorporate in my routine. Funny thing is, I have all the equipment in our basement. Rowing machine, elliptical, treadmill, weights, bands, steppers, ab wheels and other miscellaneous items. Throughout the years, I would buy equipment to get me started and every year, I would only use it for a couple of months. I played sports growing up but for whatever reason, I just stopped working out all together after college. I would occasionally go for a walk or run when I have time but to dedicate time to exercise or go to the gym was something I could not push myself to do.

This year, I wanted to get results, it is something I MUST DO. I started listening to lose weight mindset classes. I also belong to a few weight loss communities on Facebook and have enjoyed all the groups because we all have the same goal. To live a healthier life.

You may want to go to the gym and may not want to work out at home. That's okay too. I know it's more fun to do it with a group. Do what works for you.

It was tough to add exercise to my routine since I have not worked out for 15 years. I felt rusty but I was able to push through. I saw my results after 5 weeks. I was blown away. Never did I think I would get results in just 5 weeks. But I did. This got me more motivated to continue. I know it will take time and hard work to get to where I want to be, but for now I am going to celebrate the small wins.

I finally found something that is doable and having fun doing it. Never in a million years would I think I will be back to my college size again. Below are some of my before, 5 weeks and 8 weeks photos. As I continue this working out journey, I know my body will be stronger and learner as long as I don't quit on myself. This is a part of my lifestyle now and I can't wait for what's to come.

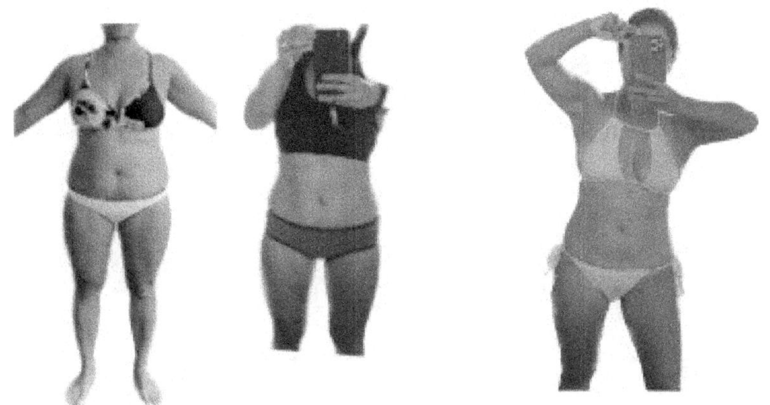

5

Fourth Habit: Meal Plan

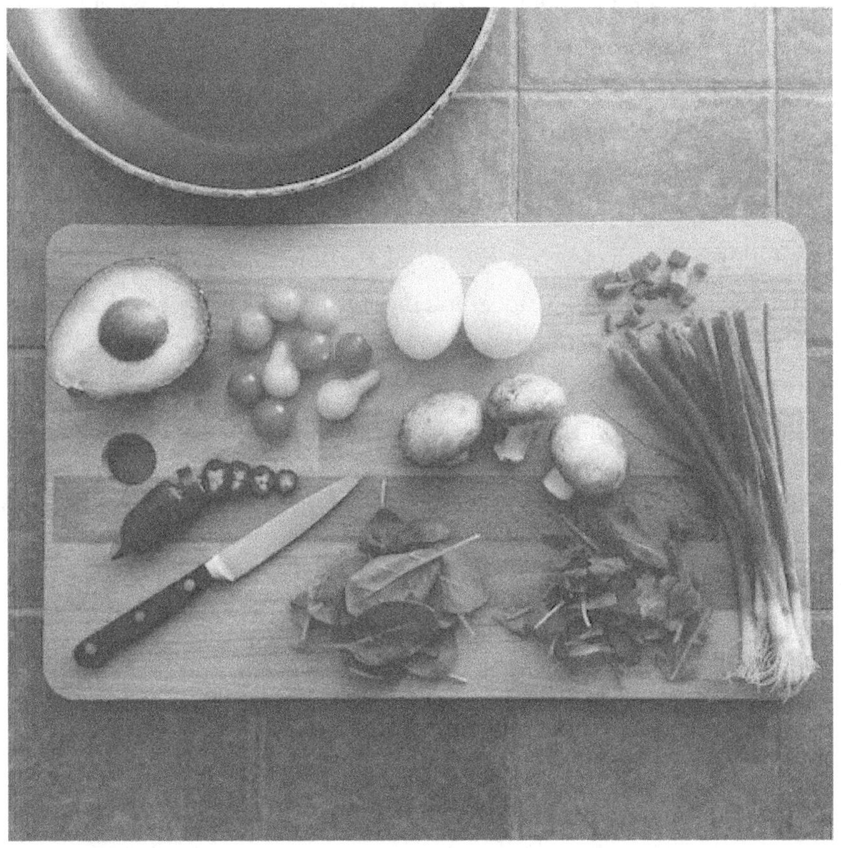

I am not the best cook, but I can follow directions. I have been exploring different types of clean eating. I need something easy and quick. Recently, a friend introduced me to the E2M Eager2cook. You can purchase it on Amazon. What I like about it. They are easy meals to make with simple ingredients. They are all healthy recipes. One of my favorites is the beef stuffed peppers or the turkey meatloaf. What I do sometimes is make a burger out of the turkey meatloaf and eat with portobello mushrooms, add avocado and a dash of spicy sauce. It is a veggie turkey burger. Try it! It is delicious. Get creative with your meal creations, mix, and match the recipes. The recipe is very flavorful. You will be amazed how easy it is to make and to follow their directions. The cookbook will also show you many different sauces or substitutions. The meals are very enjoyable. You will not be disappointed. It also shows real people's results.

When I first started clean eating, it took getting used to the recipes since it is low carbs, dairy free, no supplements and no sugar or added sugar. As I continue clean eating and trying different recipes, it is not so bad. One recommendation to consider. When you are buying your food or condiments, read the labels. Make sure it is always "NO SUGAR ADDED." I never used to pay attention until I started this new lifestyle.

So, how do you make sure you are consistent with your meal plan? You need to make sure your meals are prepared weekly so when you are hungry you can quickly grab it and heat it up.

I would cook every 3 days and would eat 2 meals a day within my eating window. Sometimes 3 meals but no more than that. I also do not snack. If I am craving sweets, I would drink flavored tea. My favorite is the Tazo - lemon glazed loaf flavor. It takes away the cravings.

I have been living this lifestyle for a year now. I did not have that much to lose but it is significant enough that I know I needed to do something. But I also know you cannot just work out and lose weight. You also need to incorporate eating healthy and other habits to see results. My recommendation is to remove any temptations from your house so you can stay on track.

Clean eating has changed my life. Is this sustainable you asked? Yes, but I do cheat once a week but only one meal per week. I can eat anything I want and have two glasses of alcohol within the 2 hours eating window. Then I go back to eating clean. It resets my mind and body and will not feel like I am deprived from not eating other foods.

I would like to provide an example of what my daily schedule looks like for 7 days. You can then incorporate your own workout plan that you enjoy and stick to it to get impressive results. I recommend doing this for 8 weeks. Then keep repeating it until you hit your weight goal. Before you start, take your measurements and weight. Then put the scale away. I know it is hard but trust me, you will be happy you did.

6

Example of Workout Plan

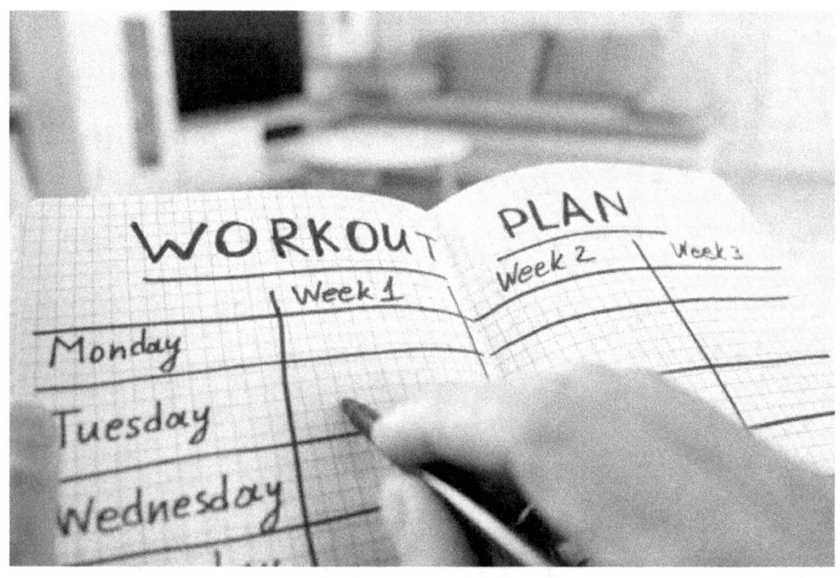

Monday, Wednesday and Friday Schedule

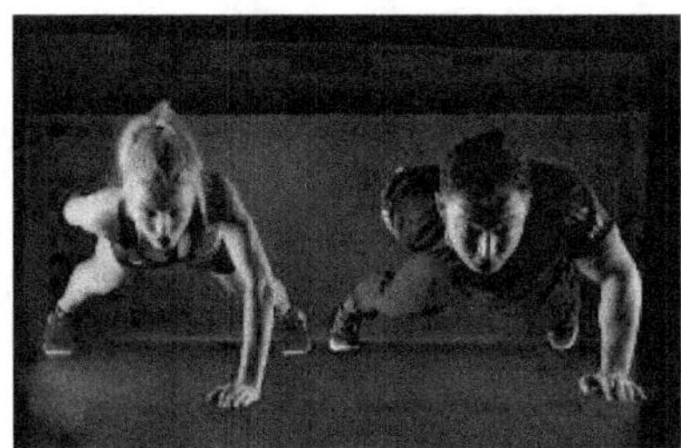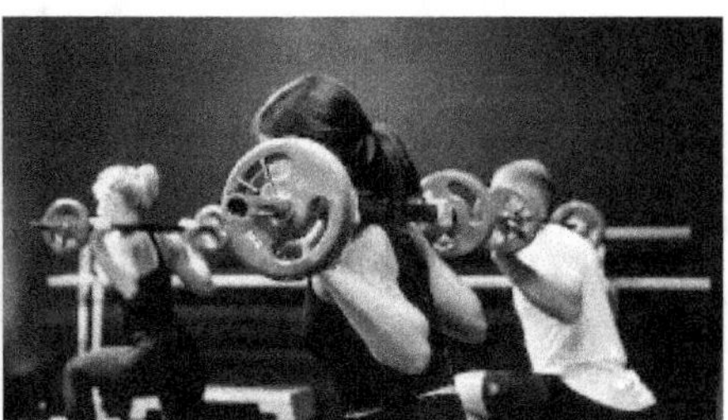

When I wake up, I would have a cup of warm apple cider vinegar (ACV) drink with a splash of mio. I would stretch then I would do my exercise (about 30 minutes). I would start with HIIT (High Intensity Interval Training) full body workout. If you are not familiar with HIIT workout - it is a short period of intense exercise until the point of exhaustion. It helps with increasing your metabolism and burns more calories. You can find some free HIIT workouts online i.e., YouTube, Instagram, or Facebook.

I would continue to drink my water until 12PM. I would have my lunch. About 2PM that is when sometimes I would crave for something. This is when I drink the Tazo flavored tea or black coffee. Then I continue to drink my water. If you have time add any 20 minutes cardio of your choice. I love to go on my treadmill or walk/run outside when the weather is nice. At 6:30 PM is when I eat my dinner. I would then continue to drink my water until I have drunk a gallon. My night cap is another warm ACV drink.

This schedule is repeated every other day.

Tuesday, Thursday and Saturday Schedule

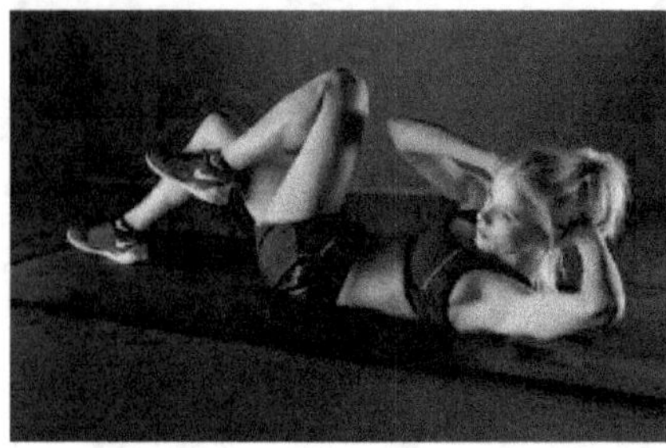 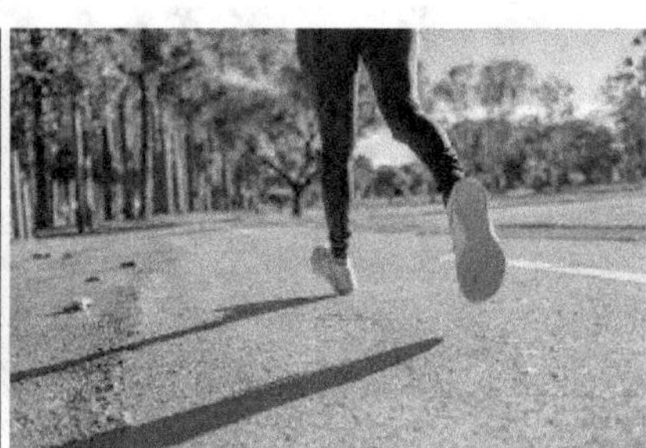

I would have a cup of warm apple cider vinegar (ACV) drink with a splash of mio. I would stretch then do my cardio exercise (about 30 minutes), again any cardio of your choice. I love kickboxing or just walking/running. I would then add abs workout or butt work out. Usually, 15 minutes each. If you are new to the exercise world like me, I would recommend checking YouTube for some free exercises or to familiarize some of the workout terms. For Butt Workouts you will hear about Donkey kicks, Bridge, Elevated Bridge, Fire Hydrant, Reverse Lunge, Chair Squat, Curtsy Lunge, Wall Squat, Standing leg Circles and many more. These are different ways to activate your legs and glutes without any equipment. For free workout, you would search abs workout or butt workout via YouTube, Instagram, or Facebook.

I would continue to drink my water until 12PM. I would have my lunch. About 2PM that is when sometimes I would crave for something. This is when I drink the Tazo flavored tea or black coffee. Then I continue to drink my water. At 6:30 PM is when I eat my dinner. I would then continue to drink my water until I have drunk a gallon. My night cap is another warm ACV drink.

This schedule is repeated every other day.

Something to keep in mind. The number on a scale is not always the best indication of your progress. So don't forget to pay attention to your measurements too.

Sunday

Rest Day

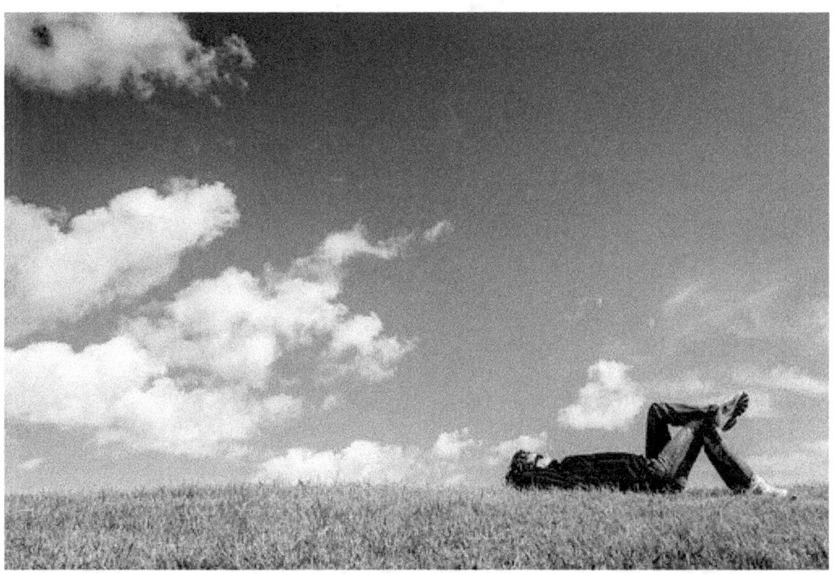

***** Every single day - I would listen to a lose weight mindset class for 15 minutes.**

That's my schedule on a weekly basis. I would then repeat it every week but would look for different HIIT or cardio workouts that I can incorporate weekly based on my schedule. Once you feel comfortable with your routine, increase your cardio workout time another 10 minutes per day until you get to an hour of cardio a day.

Once you build up your stamina and you are feeling stronger I recommend adding weight to your workout. It will help you build muscle and burn fat faster. For HIIT I use up to 10lbs and 5lbs for my abs. You can add heavier weights but it depends on what look you're going for. My goal is to lean but not bulky. The most I would use is 15lbs.

7

Mindset

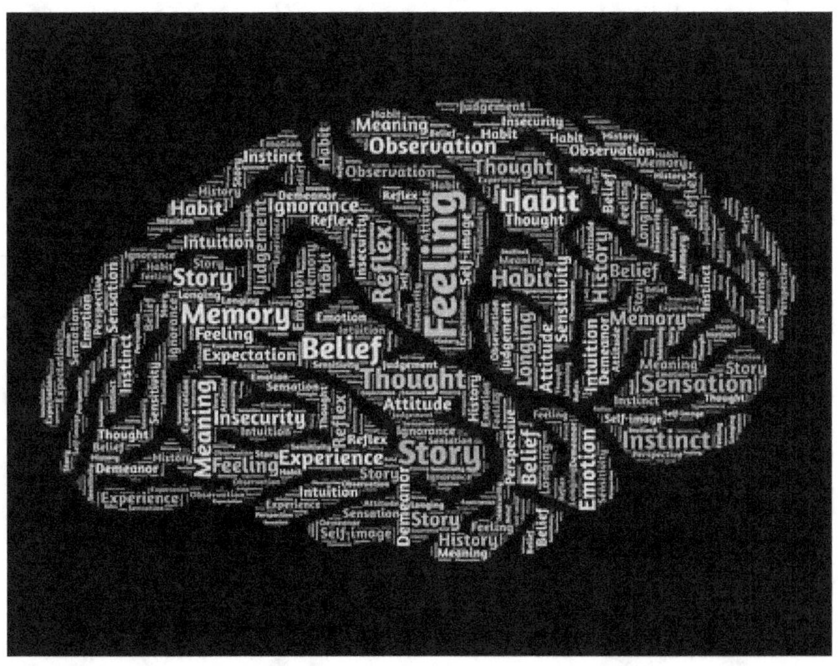

As you are aware, I have tried so many programs to help me lose weight,
but I have failed miserably until I realized that it is all in my mind. I

needed to shift my thinking. I have a purpose, which is to live longer and be there for my kids. Having my wants or purpose in my mind helped me to be able to shift my thinking and believe that I can achieve it. Without changing your mindset, your results will vary, or it could also go the other way and even put on more weight. So, you must have a definite purpose. Once your mindset shifts, you can start feeling good about yourself again and implementing these 4 habits will get you to your goal. Once you achieve your goal, you will have a better quality of life and live longer. Change your mindset and the rest will follow. Instilling your small wins will help you navigate through any challenges every day as you continue this journey.

I cannot say I did not struggle because I did. I messed up a few times. Some days I did not work out and I knew I had to do it. One thing I did not do is quit. It is all about restarting and picking back up where you left off. These habits are not about perfection. It is being able to commit, be disciplined and be consistent. If you show up for yourself, you too can get to your goal. You do not get an opportunity for a "do over" with your time. Like they said, time is nonrefundable, use it with intention. Make small goals weekly and celebrate your small wins. Try to push out of your comfort zone a little. Be uncomfortable to see what you are capable of because I promise, if I could do it, you can do it too! It is achievable. I too will continue these habits and this new lifestyle because without these daily routines, I will not be where I am today.

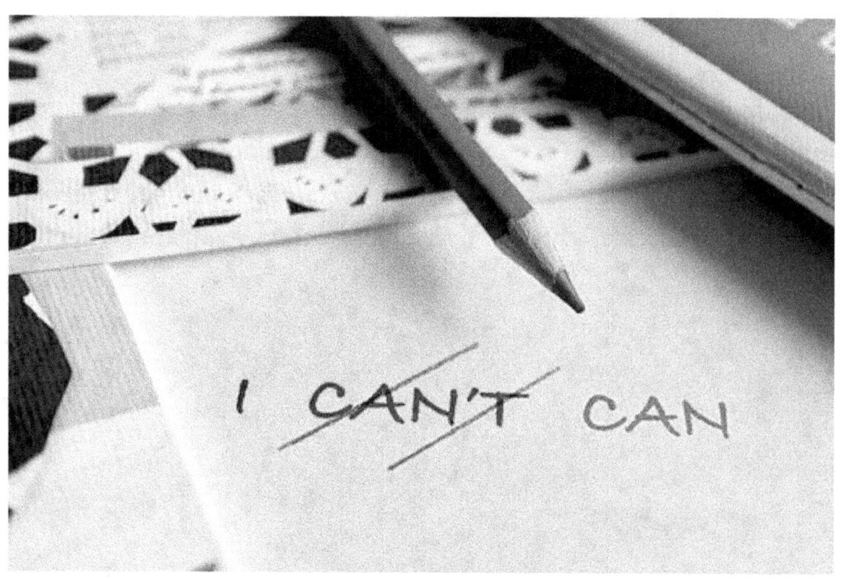

A few inspirational quotes that start my day.

1. "To change your body, you must change your mind"
2. "Decide and Commit"
3. "Your body can do anything"
4. "Celebrate the little wins"
5. "Trust the process"
6. "Think of that feeling you'll get when you reach your weight goal"
7. "When you feel like quitting, think about why you started"
8. "If it doesn't challenge you, it doesn't change you"
9. "The only person you should be better than is the person you were yesterday"
10. "If you have discipline, drive and determination - nothing is impossible"
11. "Someone busier than you is running right now"
12. "You didn't get gain all your weight in one day, you won't lose it in

one day, be patient with yourself" by Jenna Wolfe

I would read these quotes when I don't have the time to listen to a mindset class. It helps me push myself to continue the journey and not stop or fall back. I encourage you to find something that resonates with you. Read it daily and set it as a reminder why you are taking this journey.

8

It's Time for a New Beginning

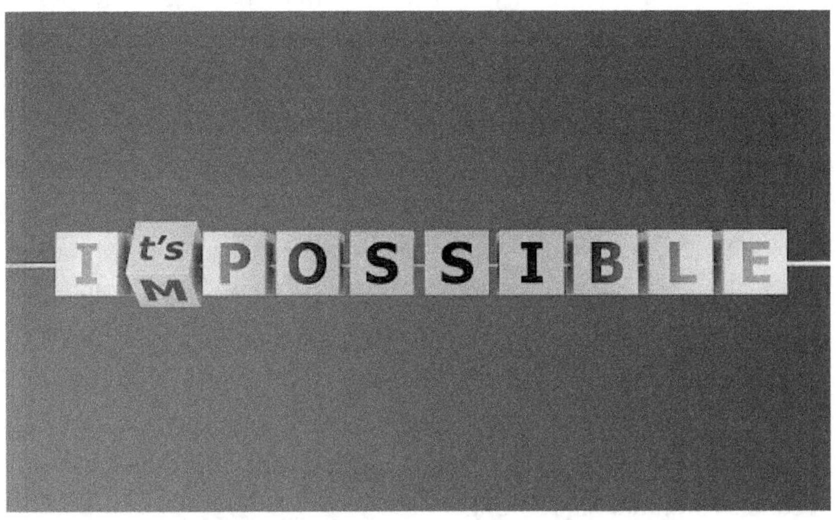

Now that you have the 4 Habits to lose weight information. You are ready to also change your life to help you get to the best shape in your life. It will be a game changer for you as soon as you incorporate these routines daily.

One thing I would say, sometimes when results do not happen right away the easiest thing to do is to give up. We forget that all your hard work will pay off if you keep pushing forward. Everyone's results are different. It could take someone 5 weeks or 3 months. Others may take a little longer, maybe because you cannot follow the routine. It is okay. If you reset, and you do not continue to fall off the wagon and completely give up. We will slip up and sometimes we may only do one or two or three of the habits but continue to push through. Something is better than nothing. It is not easy, but I recommend always resetting the next day.

This is the time for you to start fresh and make improvements in your lifestyle. It is an opportunity to work on a new challenge for yourself so get excited! You can do it too but do not overdo it. Always listen to your body. Your mind may tell you to push through but if your body is telling you to rest, there is a reason. You cannot get stronger if you fail to listen to your body.

You want to enjoy the journey and not feel like it is a chore. Once you get to your weight goal, you will be so proud you stuck to this and realize this new lifestyle is not so bad. My life forever changed and WHY NOT YOU? Prove to yourself you CAN. There will be a lot of days where you will struggle but remember your purpose it is the only way you can get back on track. The longer you do this routine the stronger you will become. You can do hard things.

9

Tips for Success

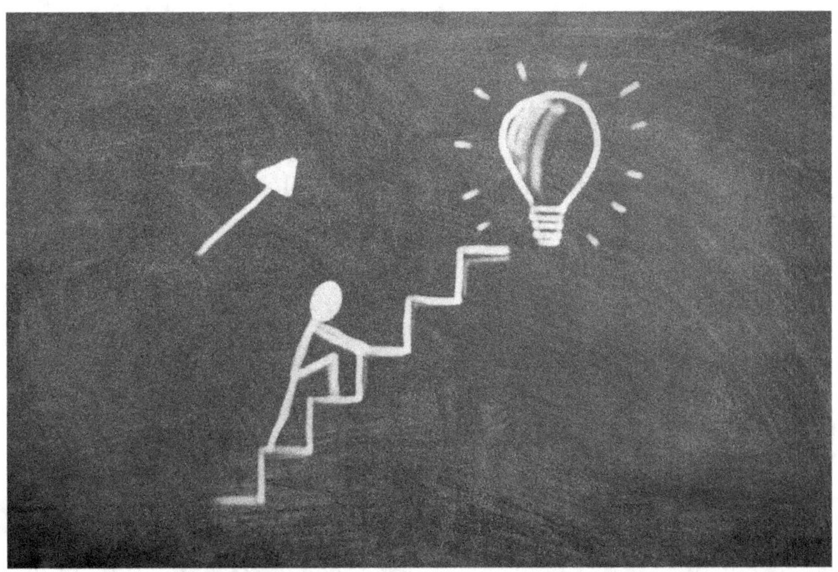

Before you begin this journey to better "YOU," take your photo, measurements, and weight. Now put the scale away and do not look at it until 8 weeks. It will only discourage you if you feel like the scale did not move. Remember, you will also be building muscles and muscles weigh more than fat.

Intermittent Fasting: Pick your 16/8 Method that works for you and stick to your eating time window.

Meal Plan: I would prepare meals on Sunday's and Wednesday's. Put them in small containers. My meal portions are: 4 to 6 oz of Protein, 1 to 2 cups of veggies and Healthy Fats (i.e., avocados, peanut butter, or nuts). I would add one cup of fruit every other week. Buy measuring cups and weigh scales if you do not already have one. I would also recommend buying a Ninja to cook your food. Less mess and easier to clean.

Exercise: Wake up early and get your workout done. Sometimes when you do it at the end of the day, something else will pop up on your schedule and you end up pushing your exercise aside. Select your workouts for the week and research free HIIT or cardio workouts. I suggest buying weights and a yoga mat. Always have water with you when you are working out.

Drink plenty of fluids: Buy a water jug with measurements to keep track of your water intake. Remember your goal is to drink a gallon of liquid daily.

Mindset: Listen to a free mindset class online daily. I would listen when I am driving or sipping my coffee or when I have some downtime. I would recommend at least 15 to 30 minutes a day. Check out Spotify or YouTube for some free Weight Loss mindset classes.

Group/Community: Find a community in the Facebook or Instagram group that will hold you accountable for your actions to ensure you are on track of your goal. You could also gather your friends and do these four habits with them. Challenge each other, do accountability check-ins, and make it fun. Share your recipes and workout plan for the day. It will help you focus on your daily task and closer to your weight goal.

One cheat meal weekly: Eat whatever you want within the two hours window of your scheduled eating window which also includes maximum two glasses of alcohol if needed (12PM - 8PM).

Pick one day Rest Day: Your body also needs a break to rejuvenate. Give it time to alleviate any muscle soreness or pain. Your muscles need time to heal or repair. So, it is important that your body gets a break to replenish your body's energy.

I would recommend checking your progress at the end of 8 weeks. Then before you start another round take another photo and measurements. Continue to do this process until you reach your weight goal.

10

Conclusion

I've been doing these 4 habits for a year now and I'm proud to say I have kept the weight off. I now have a healthier lifestyle. I know it's not easy. It's hard to eat clean all the time. These are the hurdles you must overcome to get to your goal. I struggled in the beginning. It is always hard to start but once you get going, you will be unstoppable. It's all in your mindset. Once you get that under control, your mind will give you life changing emotional benefits.

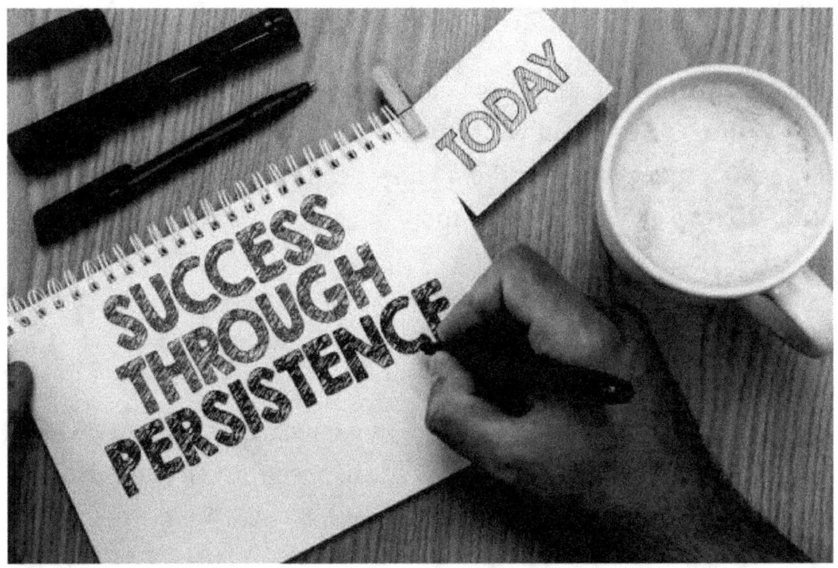

I hope you enjoyed my book. I had fun writing it. It brought back memories of my journey and my struggles. One thing I can say is whatever you are going through in your journey, I am sure I was at the same place when I was doing it. Focus on your mindset. This is doable if you are willing to make the change for yourself. I am here to tell you these 4 habits work if you incorporate it into your daily routine.

How bad do you want to change? This is up to you now. I know you can do it too. Focus on your WHYs. Whatever that is, you will be a happier person once you achieve it.

Having a plan daily or weekly will set you up for success.

I hope you continue this journey and embrace this new lifestyle. Do not go back to what you used to do. Own your goal and stick to it. You will be so proud of yourself once you accomplish what you are set to do. Imagine if you could live longer, have more energy, sleep better and happier because you finally did it.

Enjoy your journey and keep setting new goals for yourself. You are creating a new healthy lifestyle that will continue to guide you throughout the rest of your life. I know I will continue this lifestyle for years to come and hope you do too.

Kudos to you for picking up this book. That means you are ready for a change.

I believe in you. It is time to believe in yourself that you can do hard things. I cannot wait for your results to happen for you and be able to share your happiness with your loved ones.

Now, let us begin. You can do this.

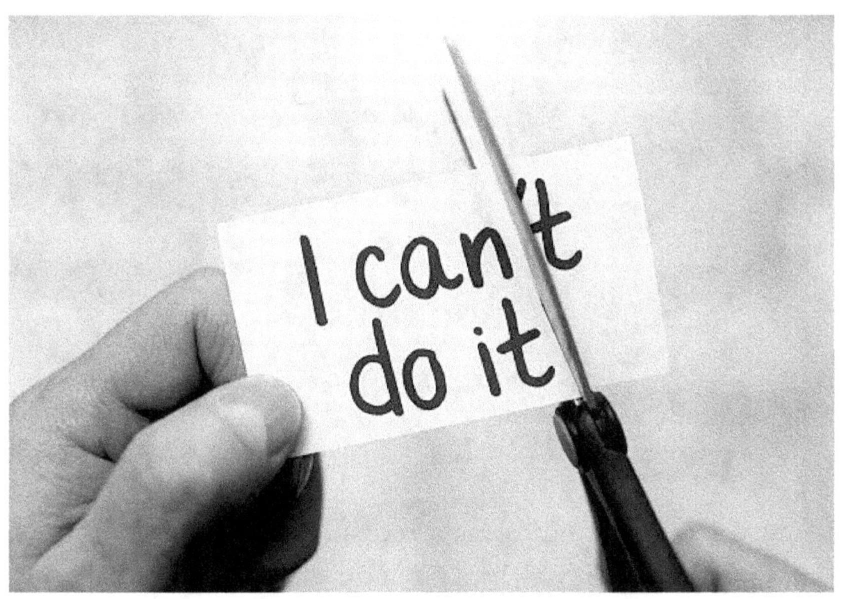

If you enjoyed this book, I would greatly appreciate it if you could leave a review for the book on Amazon.

11

Resources

Center for Disease Control and Prevention. (2022, September 19). *Losing Weight*. Centers for Disease Control and Prevention. Retrieved January 20, 2023, from https://www.cdc.gov/healthyweight/losing_w eight/getting_started.html

Mayo Clinic. (2022, October 8). *Fasting diet: Can it improve my heart health?* Retrieved January 20, 2023, from https://www.mayoclinic.org/ diseases-conditions/heart-disease/expert-answers/fasting-diet/faq-20 058334

Khan, S. (2022, September 8). *10 Proven Weight Loss Tips That Actually Work*. eMediHealth. Retrieved January 20, 2023, from https://www.em edihealth.com/nutrition/proven-weight-loss-tips

A Better Weigh Inc. (2022, August 8). *Intermittent fasting for women over 50: Benefits and tips for success*. Better Weigh Medical. Retrieved January 20, 2023, from https://betterweighmedical.com/intermittent-fasting-f or-women-over-50

Shiffer, E. (2022, March 3). *Can Drinking Water Help You Lose Weight—And How Much Should You Have Every Day?* Women's Health. Retrieved January 20, 2023, from https://www.womenshealthmag.com /health/a39265125/how-much-water-should-i-drink-to-lose-weight/

Bjarnadottir, M. A. S. (2020, December 14). *How Drinking More Water Can Help You Lose Weight.* Healthline. Retrieved January 20, 2023, from https://www.healthline.com/nutrition/drinking-water-helps-with-we ight-loss

Burnett, H. (2022, July 25). *The 12 Weight Loss Motivational Quotes You Need When You Want To Quit.* Word to Your Mother. Retrieved January 20, 2023, from https://wordtoyourmotherblog.com/weight-loss-moti vational-quotes/

Woerner, A., & Woerner, A. (2021, November 18). *Will Apple Cider Vinegar Really Help You Lose Weight?* Life by Daily Burn. https://dailybu rn.com/life/health/apple-cider-vinegar-for-weight-loss/

Jennie Casselman, E2M Chef Connect., & Chapparo, A. (2022, December 19). *Eager 2 Cook, Healthy Recipes for Healthy Living: Beef & Poultry - Kindle edition by Connect, E2M Chef, Casselman, Jennie, Chaparro, Andres. Health, Fitness & Dieting Kindle eBooks @ Amazon.com.* E2M Fitness. Retrieved January 20, 2023, from https://www.amazon.com/Eager-Co ok-Healthy-Recipes-Living-ebook/dp/B0BQLCZTN5

McIntosh, J. (2018, July 16). *Fifteen benefits of drinking water.* Retrieved January 20, 2023, from https://www.medicalnewstoday.com/articles/ 290814